Birth Story Held *for Loss*

A Guide for Reflecting on Your Fertility Experience, Miscarriage, Abortion, TFMR, Stillbirth, and Infant Loss

EMILY SOUDER, LCSW-C, PMH-C

Visit the author's website at www.emilysouder.com

This guide is not meant as a replacement for psychotherapy or working through perinatal-related topics with a professional. The reader should consult a physician or a mental health professional in matters relating to their mental health and particularly with respect to any symptoms that may require diagnosis or medical attention.

Cover and interior design by Jess Creatives

Spiral graphic by C&V Creative

Edited by Jodi Brandon

Author photo by Flaunt Your Fire

First Edition

ISBN-13: 978-1-7346309-2-3

DEDICATION

To Luna: Thank you for opening my eyes to a whole different realm of possibility—a window into another part of the human experience. I'm looking forward to continuing this partnership, even if from afar.

CONTENTS

Author's Note 7

Foreword 9

Preface 11

Introduction 15

Snails 19

An Important Note 21

Fertility Experience Reflection 23

Pregnancy or Gestation Reflection 39

Miscarriage Reflection.. 53

Abortion or Termination Reflection.................................... 67

Termination for Medical Reasons (TFMR) Reflection.................. 83

Stillbirth Pre-Birth Reflection... 99

Birth Experience Reflection

    Section 1: Starting 111

    Section 2: Progressing... 123

Section 3: Spending Time with Your Baby (or Babies) 133

Section 4: Stillbirth Reflection 143

Section 5: After 155

NICU Stay Reflection 169

Infant Loss Reflection 181

Remembering and Honoring Your Baby or Babies 195

Be in Your Body 211

Gratitude 213

Acknowledgments 215

About the Author.. 217

AUTHOR'S NOTE

Just as this space is inclusive for all birth and loss experiences, it is also inclusive of all readers regardless of their gender or the titles/terms they feel safest using. In this space, use the language you feel is the best for you.

FOREWORD

We are so sorry for your loss. No matter the type of loss, whether reproductive, early pregnancy, termination, stillbirth, or infant death, we acknowledge that the path to parenthood can be painfully complicated and offer compassion for the heartbreak you have endured.

In our experience, pregnancy and infant loss are often widely misunderstood and minimized by Western society, and we are acutely aware of the far-reaching effects that this may have on your emotional and mental well-being, your relationships, and the birth story you tell yourself and those around you.

Birth Story Held for Loss provides the opportunity for you to begin the important process of exploring and reclaiming your lived experience of love and loss through the power of story.

Story has served as a catalyst for healing and transformation for thousands of years. We believe writing and sharing your story play a significant role in how one understands, integrates, and finds meaningful connections within their experience of pregnancy and infant loss.

Your story is embodied within you; it lives in your cellular memory, mind, heart, and soul. It is colored by the myriad emotions you have and will experience, including excitement, anticipation, devastation, heartbreak, fear, deep sadness, anxiety, joy, love, grief, guilt, regret, anger, forgiveness, and hope.

It takes tremendous courage to revisit the memories and experience the full range of emotions surrounding your pregnancy and your loss(es). We encourage you to bring compassionate curiosity to your inner world as you embark on this difficult emotional journey rooted in love. Do not force anything and move slowly, with patience. Giving yourself grace and compassion, tend to yourself as you would a friend.

You may have to give yourself over to your grief and compassionately be with the waves of emotion that wash over you, even the ones that feel uncomfortable. Trust that opening yourself up is part of the process, and it is through this deeper awareness and understanding that you begin to integrate your loss(es) and reclaim your story.

This is a story of love. It is an opportunity for you to honor your broken heart, authentically express the truth of your lived experience and possibly explore your identity as a parent and your relationship with your baby. You are invited to participate in the transformational process of making meaning out of your loss.

Once you have written your story, we hope that one day you feel inspired to share it with others. Your birth story is yours to tell, and it matters, not only for honoring your baby (or babies) and integrating your lived experience, but for shattering the silence around pregnancy and infant loss and helping others realize they are not alone. We appreciate that how and when this happens will be a unique process for everyone. Whether you disclose all, some, or none of your experience to others is not a reflection of the depth of your pain or love, nor does it dishonor the life of the baby you very much wanted.

Your birth story is not fixed. It will evolve as you continue the lifelong process of making sense and meaning of your love and your loss(es.) While your life will never be the same, we believe in the healing wisdom of self-reflection and storytelling to lovingly guide you during this difficult journey of rebuilding yourself.

In love and loss,

Betsy Winter and Kiley Hanish

Return To Zero: HOPE

PREFACE

This book is intended to serve as a loving, gentle tool to assist gestating/birthing parents with processing their fertility care, pregnancy/gestation, or birth experience that resulted in a loss. This can include, but is not limited to, miscarriage, abortion, termination for medical reasons (TFMR), stillbirth, and infant loss.

The questions refer to one experience but allow for the fact that some pregnancies/gestations and births result in multiple babies. You can revisit these questions as many times as you desire to apply them to different experiences; simply use a separate journal if you have already used the lined pages within. You will also find extra lined pages at the end of each section in case you need some more space for writing.

You will notice my use of the word *baby* in some parts of the book. If that isn't a word that feels aligned for you, that is absolutely okay. Please use whichever word or words (embryo, fetus, etc.) resonate with your personal experience.

The book is divided into sections. Depending on your experiences, you might visit some of them or all of them. Some questions may not apply to you; simply skip those. As always, feel completely free to choose your path within this book. If one section resonates more than the other, take that path. You are the expert on your experience, and I trust you will do what serves you best.

- Fertility Experience Reflection: a space to reflect not only on the experience of undergoing fertility care, but also any losses experienced during that time

- Pregnancy or Gestation Reflection: appropriate for anyone who experienced that phase of parenthood, whether or not you experienced a loss during that phase
- Miscarriage Reflection: a section especially for those who experienced this type of loss during pregnancy or gestation
- Abortion or Termination Reflection: a space for those who navigated the decision to end a pregnancy or gestation and the emotions that come with that loss
- Termination for Medical Reasons (TFMR) Reflection: for those who experienced a scenario in which their physical health or their baby's (or babies') physical health shifted whether they would continue the pregnancy or gestation
- Stillbirth Pre-Birth Reflection: questions specific to the stillbirth experience that you may want to visit prior to beginning the Birth Experience Reflection
- Birth Experience Reflection: divided into five sub-sections: Starting, Progressing, Spending Time with Your Baby (or Babies), Stillbirth Reflection, and After. The sections and questions follow the progression of birth from the beginning of labor until after the baby (or babies) has been born, and they allow for variations in birth, such as cesarean section. If Stillbirth Reflection does not apply to you, move to the After section.
- NICU Stay Reflection: for families who experienced a NICU stay with their baby (or babies)
- Infant Loss Reflection: for readers whose infant passed in the hours, days, weeks, and months following birth
- Remembering and Honoring Your Baby (or Babies): No matter your type of loss experience, you may find some topics worth spending time on here, regardless of the gestational age of your embryo, fetus, or baby. This is your full permission to experience this loss as valid and real, and to reflect on it in that way.

While the case could have been made for combining the Abortion or Termination and Termination for Medical Reasons (TFMR) sections, my experience has been that there can be some important intricacies in these scenarios leading to them being best honored by having their own spaces. You are of course free to explore both sections and take what works from them for your particular story.

You can pick up and put down the guide as many times as you wish; there is no required pace. Choose the rhythm that feels right to you and set the intention to dive only into topics with which you're ready to sit for a bit. And, of course, remember to invite in lots of compassion for yourself and the stories you co-created with your baby (or babies).

INTRODUCTION

This is a space just for you. It might feel unfamiliar to have this space for your fertility care, pregnancy or gestation stories, or birth stories. Have you had space to tell your stories yet? This space was created for you to be held, here, in all the complexities and depth that come with experiencing a loss. Loss is such a personal experience, and though I am walking with you, I will not be sharing my story here. Reader, this space is completely yours.

As you already know, loss stays with you. It's an ever-shifting, moving experience. It can be heavy and crushing, leaving you breathless and unsure of who you even are anymore. At other times it can be quieter, not screaming in your ear but whispering its memories as you go about your day. Grief comes in waves, and it can swing back and forth. One moment you may be surprised to find yourself laughing at a joke, only to fall to pieces in the next moment when a familiar song starts to play. It's normal to experience grief in a fluctuating way as you move along with healing. Granting permission to feel all the things (which those around you may or may not support) is central. Find safe spaces to do this—with a therapist, dear friend, partner, or someone else whom you trust.

While all loss is individual, some types of loss feel particularly private and may have stigma attached. In these cases, most people in your life may not even be aware of what you are going through. That can feel so very lonely. Know that your experience is valid, and counts. Your loss matters. It deserves space for its story to be told.

It isn't common for friends to ask to hear how losing your baby (or babies) or having your intrauterine insemination (IUI) treatment not succeed was for you—to sit with you in your pain, confusion, grief, or shock. But your fertility care, pregnancy, and birth experiences? They're still stories. Whole, real stories. By all means, you deserve a space to explore them and tell them.

Life-changing experiences, including the painful ones, leave lasting impressions. Through them, our identities become utterly changed, breaking us open to a newness for which we are often unprepared. Fertility care, gestation or pregnancy, and birth experiences ending in loss are an example of these life-changing experiences, and that is what we are welcoming here.

Throughout our lives, we often create narratives, or stories, about things we have experienced. Our stories help our minds to make sense of things. They can both support us and limit us. Many times those stories live hidden within our minds, perhaps because we are not conscious of them or are hesitant to speak them. These thoughts can be so very tender to our souls. Plenty of times our stories leak into what we think is possible in our lives—in our parenting, in our careers, in our spirituality. Our stories can change how we relate to all the layers of our lives, and for this reason it is so very important to get curious about what we're telling ourselves.

We have an opportunity here to rewild (thanks to one of my spiritual teachers, Lindsay Mack, for using this word in a way that always brings it back to the forefront of my mind) the meaning of birth. The things that you have been told about what birth is or is not do not have a place here. The truth of what birth is to you is the only thing welcome in this space. I welcome and honor your truth and lived experience.

If you lived through a fertility treatment that wasn't effective, your loss is valid loss. Whether you experienced a miscarriage, termination, or abortion, birth is birth. Whether your baby (or babies) moved from you vaginally or via cesarean section, birth is birth. Birth ending in loss is birth. Your story is sacred. Perhaps your culture doesn't make that abundantly clear, but it is. No matter what. What story have you been telling yourself about your baby's (or babies') birth—that wedge of time between when your child spent their last moments within your body and their first moments outside of you?

Clearly, fertility, pregnancy, birth, and early parenthood stories are not always clean, straightforward, and joyful. They can be messy, complex, and mixed with pain. It serves us well to give a voice to all sides of the story, not just the parts that we feel we "should" have. It's okay to feel shock and calm, grief and awe. This book creates a path for you to explore your story, to turn it over and examine it as you would a shell on a sandy beach or a rock on a mossy path. Be curious. Find a beautiful journal in which you can pen your responses, or record them here. You may choose to share your journaling with others, or you may not. That's up to you.

I invite you to write down your fertility, pregnancy or gestation, and/or birth story in its entirety, either together with your responses to these prompts or elsewhere. You can begin the story wherever feels right to you, even if it begins months or years before the actual experience. Authentically reviewing the details can help you process the event and will also document information that might otherwise get lost in your memory.

After sharing space with so many clients who benefit from putting a voice to their story, I believe even more deeply in the value of intentionally going within and seeing what's there. As some parents may have navigated hospital time with their baby (or babies), I have included a special section for parents who experienced a NICU stay with their little one(s). My work with families has shown me how much some extra reflection and compassion around that time can help with healing. Also, you will find an invitation to reconnect with your physical body at the end of the book. While my intention is to keep that part of you involved throughout the questions, I want to make extra sure that you touch base with it before finishing up. There can be so many complex feelings related to your body after a loss, and it makes sense that your relationship with your own body may need attention and healing as well.

It goes without saying that the questions I offer will not touch all areas of your story, but my hope is that they will open a pathway for you to explore. Follow the questions where they lead. Be brave (and also gentle). Look into yourself and tune in. Hear the voice asking for a listening ear.

You have a story to tell. Let's walk this path together. I invite you to leave judgment at the door. Get comfy, and let's begin.

SNAILS?

For those of you familiar with *Birth Story Brave* and *Birth Story Brave, Reimagined*, you may remember that on the covers are photos of snails. While this book is different in many ways, I wanted to keep the spiral, which beckons that inward reflection. You might recognize the spiral inside these pages from the interior of the original *Birth Story Brave*.

When I was thinking about and planning the first *Birth Story Brave*, snail shells and snails seemed to follow me around—way more than enough to catch my attention. I've always liked snails, but I'd only seen a handful of them in person over the course of my lifetime. All of a sudden, upon starting my original book, they were everywhere: shells upon shells that had washed up on the beach, tiny friends visiting our garden, and even on my front porch as I walked through my front door.

I am often one to look to animals for messages when they appear so purposely in my life, and this situation was no different. I read about snails and the reminder they give to slow down. I came back to that message again and again throughout the publishing of *Birth Story Brave*. Slow down, let it happen, don't rush it.

The shells' physical shape also seems to carry even deeper meaning, and some believe they can represent the life cycle, fertility, and change. Even without these meanings attached, there is something about that beautiful shape. It seems to invite us to be still and reflect. It beckons us to both go inward and outward, flowing, expanding and contracting. This is exactly what we're doing here with our stories.

So, the spirals and snail messengers still needed a place in this book. Let them remind you as well to take it slow and pause, following the spiral to that tender center part of yourself.

AN IMPORTANT NOTE

This book is not meant to replace psychotherapy or working through fertility, pregnancy, gestation, birth-related, or grief-related topics with a professional. However, it can of course be used as a tool within the context of such work.

It's healthy, and so very helpful, to receive professional support if you have experienced a loss. Also, if you have symptoms of depression and/ or anxiety, please don't hesitate to seek professional help with working through it. If you notice that journaling about your experience triggers a strong reaction that feels scary to you, don't be afraid or embarrassed to ask for help. More people have been there than you know. Return To Zero: HOPE (www.rtzhope.org), Stillborn and Infant Loss Support (www.bornintosilence.org), and Postpartum Support International (www.postpartum.net) are great places to start looking for resources.

FERTILITY EXPERIENCE REFLECTION

Fertility care experiences intensify the emotional experience of starting or growing a family. With high highs and low lows, fertility treatments can feel like a full-blown rollercoaster ride of hope, followed by grief, followed by hope. The whiplash of this can leave you feeling bruised, tender, and so very worn. And, of course, outcomes of such experiences vary widely. There are ripple effects to your relationships, your sense of self, and the amount of "extra" thoughts and responsibilities you can carry from day to day. This is your space to explore how it was for you.

Whether or not loss was part of your fertility care story, grief may have surfaced nonetheless. In the pages that follow, spend time where reflection is needed, and leave the rest.

One

Where does your fertility experience begin? How prepared were you for what was to come?

_____

_____

_____

_____

_____

_____

_____

_____

_____

_____

_____

_____

_____

_____

_____

_____

Two

Who went through this experience with you? Was there a partner involved in this process? Did you have friends on whom you leaned? What were the helpful or unhelpful parts of having these particular people along for the experience?

_____

_____

_____

_____

_____

_____

_____

_____

_____

_____

_____

_____

_____

Three

Were your providers—both their overall energy and their actions—how you expected them to be? Sometimes relationships with our providers can be the source of tremendous support; other times they highlight what we wish was present. In what ways did your providers assist you? In what ways, if any, did you wish you were supported differently?

_____

_____

_____

_____

_____

_____

_____

_____

_____

_____

_____

_____

_____

_____

Four

When entering into fertility care, you may have had many life changes to make and thoughts to wrestle with. The changes could have been financial or lifestyle-related, or you may have had some belief systems in place that you needed to come to terms with. What did you need to sacrifice to begin the fertility care process? What things did you need to accept? What things did you need to release?

_____

_____

_____

_____

_____

_____

_____

_____

_____

_____

_____

_____

_____

_____

_____

Five

Continuing from the previous question, are there things you have yet to accept about your fertility experience? These can be thoughts, beliefs, circumstances, or something else. Hold these things gently and with curiosity, not needing to force them to be different than they were.

_____

_____

_____

_____

_____

_____

_____

_____

_____

_____

_____

_____

_____

_____

Six

Losses come in many forms—for example, periodic losses of hope, or the loss experienced when a procedure isn't effective. What losses did you experience during your fertility experience? Were these losses acknowledged as you were going through them? How might they have been honored differently?

_____

_____

_____

_____

_____

_____

_____

_____

_____

_____

_____

_____

_____

_____

Seven

What kept you going during the challenging times? On whom or what did you rely? For example, maybe there was a podcast or support group that gave you hope when you had none left, or a friend who was great at listening.

_____

_____

_____

_____

_____

_____

_____

_____

_____

_____

_____

_____

_____

Eight

What unexpected things did you encounter throughout your fertility experience? Was there something you learned about yourself or perhaps a partner?

_____

_____

_____

_____

_____

_____

_____

_____

_____

_____

_____

_____

_____

_____

_____

_____

_____

Nine

Processing our emotions and experience takes time. With healing and allowing our emotions to move, things can happen bit by bit, rather than all at once. What amount of gentleness can you invite into your story or around your experience? Does forgiveness, of yourself or others, have a place here?

_____

_____

_____

_____

_____

_____

_____

_____

_____

_____

_____

_____

_____

_____

Ten

Does your fertility story have a title? The words you choose are ones you don't need to share with anyone unless you want to. There are truly no rules when it comes to this part. If you can't think of a title, how would you describe your story? You can make a list of words; let them cover all the bases. Some may appear to be opposites existing at the very same time (which is normal and very human).

From here, find which section supports you best. If you are not moving to a pregnancy/gestation section, you may find the section "Remembering and Honoring Your Baby (or Babies)" supportive to you as well. Whether or not you describe your loss as a "baby," you get to see if the questions resonate with you. Take what works and skip the rest. If you need more space for journaling, don't forget there are some extra lined pages at the end of each section.

Other Thoughts

_____

_____

_____

_____

_____

_____

_____

_____

_____

_____

_____

_____

_____

_____

_____

_____

Other Thoughts

_____

_____

_____

_____

_____

_____

_____

_____

_____

_____

_____

_____

_____

_____

_____

_____

_____

Other Thoughts

_____

_____

_____

_____

_____

_____

_____

_____

_____

_____

_____

_____

_____

_____

_____

PREGNANCY OR GESTATION REFLECTION

So much change blows in when a baby is (or babies are) conceived. Some people feel physical changes quite early; others have subtler cues that their body is working on something—building a new life—behind the scenes. This section is for reflecting on the time of the growing, whether you experienced your loss during this time, or later. Skip the questions that do not apply to you and find your next landing place within these pages. As always, hold yourself gently. Take time to step away if needed. You can always return later.

Just as with your birth experience, your pregnancy or gestation might not have been anything like you imagined. This can be due to health challenges, life circumstances, decisions you needed to make, or something else entirely. On the other hand, the pregnancy experience may have been absolutely fulfilling or joyful. And don't forget there is lots of room for experiences in between. Never forget that as humans we can hold such emotional complexity, which can include all different feelings, even if they seem conflicting.

Is reviewing your pregnancy something that would serve you? Spending some extra time honoring that period may be an important part of sitting with your loss experience(s). There is no need to rush forward; spend as much time with this topic as you need. Jot down things you know you would like to remember, feelings you never expected, or memories that are particularly poignant.

One

Where does your family-building story start? Was this expected? Unexpected? How, if at all, did you plan for it?

_____

_____

_____

_____

_____

_____

_____

_____

_____

_____

_____

_____

_____

_____

_____

_____

_____

Two

What was unexpected about your pregnancy or gestation? What were
the biggest surprises? For example, did you learn something about how
your body responds to preparing for or carrying a pregnancy or gestation?

_____

_____

_____

_____

_____

_____

_____

_____

_____

_____

_____

_____

_____

_____

Three

What were the biggest joys? Challenges? Dreams and hopes? Fears? Our feelings can be all over the place during this time. See what you can do to identify all of these, even if some of them feel conflicting.

_____

_____

_____

_____

_____

_____

_____

_____

_____

_____

_____

_____

_____

_____

_____

Four

Who or what were your most cherished supports during pregnancy or gestation? Were there any supports you wished you had, but didn't?

_____

_____

_____

_____

_____

_____

_____

_____

_____

_____

_____

_____

_____

_____

_____

_____

Five

It is understandable to want things to have been different in your pregnancy or gestation. Take a moment to reflect on any regrets or what-ifs you may have from your experience: actions taken or not taken, thoughts you may have had, things you said or did not say. Gently becoming aware of these is a good place to start. Take a moment here to write down anything coming up for you.

Hold these thoughts and ideas with compassion. When you're ready, experimenting with ways to release or move these through your system—whether with movement, visualization, meditation, or some other practice—is a great next step. It's okay if they're not ready to move along just yet. Now might feel like a good time to place a hand over your heart or belly, seeing what is ready to move—either by way of tears, breath, words, or something else. There is no need to force this.

_____

_____

_____

_____

_____

_____

_____

_____

_____

_____

Six

Reflect on your relationship to your body during pregnancy or gestation. How did it feel? How much trust did you feel toward your body?

_____

_____

_____

_____

_____

_____

_____

_____

_____

_____

_____

_____

_____

_____

_____

Seven

Reflect on your attachment to your baby (or babies). What did it feel like to carry them? What was your relationship like? There is a huge range in how attached people feel to their babies at this point; some people feel very connected right away, and others take more time.

_____

_____

_____

_____

_____

_____

_____

_____

_____

_____

_____

_____

_____

_____

_____

_____

Eight

Overall, what words would you use to describe your pregnancy or gestation? You will see this message many times throughout this book: The words on the list might not all feel positive—and that is okay, very much allowed, and common. Seeing the experience in its fullness and wholeness is an embracing of your humanness.

_____

_____

_____

_____

_____

_____

_____

_____

_____

_____

_____

_____

_____

From here, when you're ready, move to whichever section best describes the experience on which you are reflecting. Remember there is no prescribed timeline, so do this when it feels healing and aligned. If you need more space for journaling, don't forget there are some extra lined pages at the end of each section.

Other Thoughts

_____

_____

_____

_____

_____

_____

_____

_____

_____

_____

_____

_____

_____

_____

_____

Other Thoughts

_____

_____

_____

_____

_____

_____

_____

_____

_____

_____

_____

_____

_____

_____

_____

Other Thoughts

MISCARRIAGE REFLECTION

If you have not yet completed the previous section, make sure to see if any of the questions apply to you or would support you before you move through this section.

In this section, there is space for you to reflect and share the story of your miscarriage experience. The ending of your pregnancy is something that you are allowed to take time to grieve. You may or may not have shared about your pregnancy with any or many people, and that can make the grieving experience feel lonely. As always, be gentle with yourself. Move through questions as you feel ready, being brave but never pushing yourself too far.

One

When did you become aware that your pregnancy or gestation story was shifting? What were your initial reactions?

_____

_____

_____

_____

_____

_____

_____

_____

_____

_____

_____

_____

_____

_____

_____

Two

Through what phases did your miscarriage story move? What was your body's physical process? What was your emotional process? There can be spiritual and social components as well.

_____

_____

_____

_____

_____

_____

_____

_____

_____

_____

_____

_____

_____

_____

_____

_____

_____

Three

What are the different locations where your miscarriage took place? Did these feel like safe and supportive spaces to be in? Who was with you? Reflect on their presence. What did it make possible, and what may it have made more challenging?

_____

_____

_____

_____

_____

_____

_____

_____

_____

_____

_____

_____

_____

_____

_____

Four

What, if any, coping skills did you rely on to get through times of grief, uncertainty, or confusion? Was there anything you tried that felt particularly grounding or steadying? Did you feel numb or emotionless at times? All these different waves of emotion can be typical ways of moving through the loss experience.

_____

_____

_____

_____

_____

_____

_____

_____

_____

_____

_____

_____

_____

_____

_____

Five

Did you feel as though you were given or took the space you needed to grieve? Sometimes these losses can feel so very private and isolating, and not everyone feels that they have full permission to experience all their feelings. This loss is valid, and it counts.

_____

_____

_____

_____

_____

_____

_____

_____

_____

_____

_____

_____

_____

_____

Six

What were your feelings about the professionals who supported you before, during, and after your miscarriage? Which types of support were helpful? Which types of support were not helpful? What made things helpful or unhelpful?

_____

_____

_____

_____

_____

_____

_____

_____

_____

_____

_____

_____

_____

_____

_____

Seven

Did you require any medical procedures related to your miscarriage? What was the environment like where you experienced your procedure? Did you feel supported? How did the environment feel to your physical body?

_____

_____

_____

_____

_____

_____

_____

_____

_____

_____

_____

_____

_____

_____

Eight

During recovery, who was around you? Which types of support felt really good, and which didn't? Were you missing anyone specific, or any type of support?

_____

_____

_____

_____

_____

_____

_____

_____

_____

_____

_____

_____

_____

_____

From here, when you are ready, you may wish to move on to the Remembering and Honoring Your Baby (or Babies) section. You may find some questions that are important for your healing process. If you need more space for journaling, don't forget there are some extra lined pages at the end of each section.

Other Thoughts

_____

_____

_____

_____

_____

_____

_____

_____

_____

_____

_____

_____

_____

_____

_____

_____

Other Thoughts

_____

_____

_____

_____

_____

_____

_____

_____

_____

_____

_____

_____

_____

_____

_____

_____

_____

Other Thoughts

_____

_____

_____

_____

_____

_____

_____

_____

_____

_____

_____

_____

_____

_____

_____

_____

_____

_____

ABORTION OR TERMINATION REFLECTION

The personal choices we must make are, without a doubt, not always easy. Sometimes, we may even wish someone else would step in and tell us the "right" thing to do. But that's just it: "Right" is relative. What the right thing is for one person or family will be different from what is right for their neighbor, their cousin, or the person who cuts their hair. The choice that was safe, healthy, and best for you is honored here. Full stop. I invite you to leave what is right for everyone else at the door.

One

Where does your story begin? When or how did you discover your pregnancy or gestation?

_____

_____

_____

_____

_____

_____

_____

_____

_____

_____

_____

_____

_____

_____

_____

Two

What were your initial thoughts about your pregnancy or gestation? Did these thoughts change over time or remain the same? Note that there can be thoughts that seem to conflict with one another. For example, you might have wished things were different while also being grateful for your options.

_____

_____

_____

_____

_____

_____

_____

_____

_____

_____

_____

_____

_____

_____

_____

Three

Walk gently throughout your decision-making process around abortion or termination. Who supported you throughout this decision? What was helpful while you waded through? What was unhelpful?

_____

_____

_____

_____

_____

_____

_____

_____

_____

_____

_____

_____

_____

_____

_____

Four

When you were carrying your pregnancy or gestation, did your mind stretch into the future at all to imagine what life might look like? What did you imagine? Was there fear, doubt, or perhaps curiosity? What feelings or thoughts, if any, are ready to move or be released?

_____

_____

_____

_____

_____

_____

_____

_____

_____

_____

_____

_____

_____

_____

_____

_____

Five

Did you feel supported by your providers? What did they do or not do? Did you feel seen, heard, and held? Reflect on different experiences if you had multiple providers.

_____

_____

_____

_____

_____

_____

_____

_____

_____

_____

_____

_____

_____

_____

_____

Six

How easy was it for you to access the care you needed? Did you need to arrange for childcare, travel, or other things? Do you find yourself wishing anything had been different about this aspect of your care?

_____

_____

_____

_____

_____

_____

_____

_____

_____

_____

_____

_____

_____

_____

_____

_____

_____

Seven

What feels important to release or put a voice to about your abortion?
In other words, is there a feeling that hasn't been shared that needs to
be spoken? What would it say?

_____

_____

_____

_____

_____

_____

_____

_____

_____

_____

_____

_____

_____

_____

Eight

What supports were present for you during your recovery? Who showed up for you? Who do you wish had shown up? What were the ways in which you were supported that showed love and caring?

_____

_____

_____

_____

_____

_____

_____

_____

_____

_____

_____

_____

_____

_____

_____

_____

Nine

It is common for those experiencing a termination to question their decision or have complex feelings about it. Is there any sort of forgiveness being asked for? Or perhaps even an opening to the possibility of forgiveness? This might be something involving another person, or it could even be with yourself. No need to force anything here; just an invitation to be curious.

_____

_____

_____

_____

_____

_____

_____

_____

_____

_____

_____

_____

_____

Ten

What is your story called? What main words or phrases would you choose to describe living through your abortion or termination story from the very start? If nothing comes to you right away, let it sit for a bit. There's no rush here. You have plenty of space and time.

_____

_____

_____

_____

_____

_____

_____

_____

_____

_____

_____

_____

_____

_____

Every story is different. You may wish to turn to the Remembering and Honoring Your Baby (or Babies) section, as there might be additional things that you wish to unpack there. It's also possible that your reflection feels complete (for now) after finishing this section. If you need more space for journaling, don't forget there are some extra lined pages at the end of each section.

Other Thoughts

_____

_____

_____

_____

_____

_____

_____

_____

_____

_____

_____

_____

_____

_____

_____

_____

Other Thoughts

Other Thoughts

_____

_____

_____

_____

_____

_____

_____

_____

_____

_____

_____

_____

_____

_____

_____

_____

TERMINATION FOR MEDICAL REASONS (TFMR) REFLECTION

There are times when we need to make impossible choices, ones that make us feel raw with doubt and grief. These choices can be absolutely devastating. This section is a place for those who made the decision to terminate a pregnancy or gestation after learning about a baby's (or babies') medical condition or a situation in which your health, as the carrier, was at risk. It's a chance for you to say how this made you feel, name who was around you, and give a voice to all sides of your story. This space is for holding you.

One

Where does your family-building story begin? How did it feel to learn about your pregnancy or gestation?

Two

What are your most cherished memories from your pregnancy or gestation before any concerns arose?

_____

_____

_____

_____

_____

_____

_____

_____

_____

_____

_____

_____

_____

_____

_____

Three

At what point in your story did concerns arise? How were they shared with you? Were they shared with compassion? If you had been the provider, how might you have shared concerns differently? What did you need to hear? It's okay to say those words to yourself now.

_____

_____

_____

_____

_____

_____

_____

_____

_____

_____

_____

_____

_____

_____

Four

In what ways were your options shared with you? Did you feel they were well presented? See if there is a need to gently reflect on the element of choice here, such as whether you had—or felt you had—a choice.

_____

_____

_____

_____

_____

_____

_____

_____

_____

_____

_____

_____

_____

_____

_____

_____

Five

Did you feel supported by your providers? What did they do or not do? Did you feel seen, heard, and held?

_____

_____

_____

_____

_____

_____

_____

_____

_____

_____

_____

_____

_____

_____

_____

Six

When it comes to the time of the termination itself (whether surgical or not), did you feel supported? What type of termination did you experience? In what ways could you tell you were valued? In what ways was it hard to tell?

_____

_____

_____

_____

_____

_____

_____

_____

_____

_____

_____

_____

_____

_____

_____

Seven

What did you learn about yourself during this experience? Are there any personal qualities that you didn't know you had? Who was moving through this experience with you? Did you learn anything about them?

_____

_____

_____

_____

_____

_____

_____

_____

_____

_____

_____

_____

_____

_____

_____

_____

Eight

What supports were present for you during your recovery? Who showed up for you? Who do you wish had shown up?

_____

_____

_____

_____

_____

_____

_____

_____

_____

_____

_____

_____

_____

_____

_____

_____

_____

Nine

Was your grief respected and honored? Did you have a place to share your story?

_____

_____

_____

_____

_____

_____

_____

_____

_____

_____

_____

_____

_____

_____

Ten

What main words or phrases would you use to describe living through your loss experience? What is your story called? If nothing comes to you right away, let it sit for a bit. There's no rush here. You have plenty of space and time.

_____

_____

_____

_____

_____

_____

_____

_____

_____

_____

_____

_____

_____

_____

If it fits with how you feel about your pregnancy or gestation, you may wish to turn to the Remembering and Honoring Your Baby (or Babies) section. There might be additional things that you wish to unpack there. If you need more space for journaling, don't forget there are some extra lined pages at the end of each section.

Other Thoughts

_____

_____

_____

_____

_____

_____

_____

_____

_____

_____

_____

_____

_____

_____

_____

_____

_____

Other Thoughts

Other Thoughts

STILLBIRTH PRE-BIRTH REFLECTION

This section will not apply to every stillbirth experience. Yet, this space needed to be included for those who began labor with the knowledge that their baby (or babies) would be stillborn. Starting with the Pregnancy or Gestation Reflection section will allow you to capture the beginning of your story.

One

Where does your pregnancy or gestation story shift? In other words, at what point did you have concerns or were concerns brought to your attention about your baby (or babies)?

Two

What are your most cherished memories from the time before any concerns arose?

_____

_____

_____

_____

_____

_____

_____

_____

_____

_____

_____

_____

_____

_____

Three

How did your provider deliver information about your baby (or babies) to you? While hearing your baby has (or babies have) passed is absolutely never something you want to hear from someone, was the way your provider communicated with you helpful or unhelpful? Imagine you were in the role of your provider. What may you have done differently? It's okay to say the words to yourself that you needed to hear.

_____

_____

_____

_____

_____

_____

_____

_____

_____

_____

_____

_____

_____

_____

Four

Who was around you when you learned about your baby's (or babies')
health status? What did their energy feel like to you? Was it helpful to
have them present?

_____

_____

_____

_____

_____

_____

_____

_____

_____

_____

_____

_____

_____

_____

Five

Moving into your birth experience, how did the birth professionals around you interact with you? Did you feel respected and supported? Did you feel your baby was (or babies were) respected?

_____

_____

_____

_____

_____

_____

_____

_____

_____

_____

_____

_____

_____

_____

In the next section, we will transition to exploring your birth experience. If you need to pause here, please take time to do so. You have full autonomy about how and when you move through these questions. If you already notice some energy or emotion that is ready to shift a bit, breathe. Without forcing it out or in a certain direction, start with giving it permission to exist and then observe as you allow it to move. If you need more space for journaling, don't forget there are some extra lined pages at the end of each section.

Other Thoughts

_____

_____

_____

_____

_____

_____

_____

_____

_____

_____

_____

_____

_____

_____

_____

Other Thoughts

_____

_____

_____

_____

_____

_____

_____

_____

_____

_____

_____

_____

_____

_____

_____

_____

Other Thoughts

BIRTH EXPERIENCE REFLECTION
SECTION 1: STARTING

This is the very beginning of your birth story. This is where pregnancy or gestation nears an end and birth begins its whisper or its roar. All types of birth are welcome here. For some readers, this may be a time of great sadness, while for others a loss may not have occurred yet. This is your story, and it will intertwine with your baby's story (or babies' stories). Let's start the process of telling it.

One

This is the moment when you knew for sure: I'm going to birth my baby (or babies) today—or in the coming days, if your story lasts longer. Close your eyes and remember. What was your first thought upon being induced, when you realized that was a "real" contraction, or when you woke up on the day of your scheduled cesarean section? Maybe the birth took you by complete surprise, and you didn't have much time to think ahead. Wherever your story starts is okay. Reflect on it now.

_____

_____

_____

_____

_____

_____

_____

_____

_____

_____

_____

_____

_____

Two

At the beginning of your birth story, what hopes were you bringing into this experience with you? What fears were there? There may be plenty of times when mixed feelings or seemingly conflicting feelings arise throughout your story. That makes you so very human.

_____

_____

_____

_____

_____

_____

_____

_____

_____

_____

_____

_____

_____

_____

_____

_____

_____

Three

How did you feel about your body and what it was about to experience? Were you feeling strong and capable? Uncertain? Weak? What
was your body telling you?

_____

_____

_____

_____

_____

_____

_____

_____

_____

_____

_____

_____

_____

_____

_____

_____

Four

What did the environment around you feel like? Peaceful? Chaotic? Energized? Did this support you throughout this experience? How did it support you, and how was it unhelpful?

_____

_____

_____

_____

_____

_____

_____

_____

_____

_____

_____

_____

_____

_____

Five

How did you cope with any feelings of uncertainty? Did you rely on those around you? An inner mantra? Meditation? Distraction?

_____

_____

_____

_____

_____

_____

_____

_____

_____

_____

_____

_____

_____

_____

_____

_____

Six

Close your eyes and picture yourself at this part in your story. What image comes to mind? It doesn't have to be a snapshot of the actual event. Maybe you see something different, like an animal or colors. What does this represent to you?

_____

_____

_____

_____

_____

_____

_____

_____

_____

_____

_____

_____

_____

Seven

Look over the pages you have written in this section. Have any themes emerged? Place your hand over your heart and take several deep breaths. What do you notice? What, if anything, can you release or forgive? If you sense any judgment, give yourself permission to let it go, and exhale. Invite in love and understanding—the kind you would extend to your very best friend.

_____

_____

_____

_____

_____

_____

_____

_____

_____

_____

_____

_____

_____

_____

Other Thoughts

_____

_____

_____

_____

_____

_____

_____

_____

_____

_____

_____

_____

_____

_____

_____

Other Thoughts

_____

_____

_____

_____

_____

_____

_____

_____

_____

_____

_____

_____

_____

_____

_____

_____

Other Thoughts

_____

_____

_____

_____

_____

_____

_____

_____

_____

_____

_____

_____

_____

_____

_____

_____

BIRTH EXPERIENCE REFLECTION
SECTION 2: PROGRESSING

The journey has intensified. You're in labor, possibly working through strong contractions, and not knowing how long this will continue. Or maybe you're about to go into an operating room, uncertain of what's ahead. There are so many possibilities for what your story looks like here. Every person's story is different. However your story is unfolding, this section covers everything up to the point of your baby (or babies) being outside of your body.

One

You are in the midst of your birth journey. What are your senses saying to you at this point in the story? Remember what you heard, smelled, saw. Recall touches that felt good and didn't feel so good.

_____

_____

_____

_____

_____

_____

_____

_____

_____

_____

_____

_____

_____

_____

Two

Who is around you? What is their energy like? What is the general feeling of the environment around you? Are you aware of things outside of yourself? It's very possible that you may have been too focused on the task at hand to be paying any attention to external qualities. In either case, reflect on your inner environment as well. Is it quiet? Peaceful? Buzzing?

_____

_____

_____

_____

_____

_____

_____

_____

_____

_____

_____

_____

_____

_____

Three

Did anything happen at this point that you didn't like? Things that felt wrong or out of alignment? Especially if you had developed a carefully constructed birth plan—and even if you didn't—anything different from what you had envisioned might not sit well. For example, did you feel pressured to stay in one position when you wanted to walk around, or did you not have the options you wanted for pain control?

_____

_____

_____

_____

_____

_____

_____

_____

_____

_____

_____

_____

_____

_____

Four

Were there any moments during this time when you felt particularly proud of yourself? Take time to recognize your courage and strength, even if it feels a bit odd or out of place to consider that part of your story.

_____

_____

_____

_____

_____

_____

_____

_____

_____

_____

_____

_____

_____

_____

Five

Reflect on the providers who supported you through your birth experience. Was their support what you needed? How did it help or hinder your experience?

_____

_____

_____

_____

_____

_____

_____

_____

_____

_____

_____

_____

_____

_____

Six

Is there anything that feels unfinished? Think about some of the things you listed for question Three. This is also a place where it may be helpful to experiment with inviting in self-compassion, self-love, or perhaps even forgiveness. Again, no forcing is necessary.

_____

_____

_____

_____

_____

_____

_____

_____

_____

_____

_____

_____

_____

_____

Other Thoughts

Other Thoughts

_____

_____

_____

_____

_____

_____

_____

_____

_____

_____

_____

_____

_____

_____

_____

_____

Other Thoughts

_____

_____

_____

_____

_____

_____

_____

_____

_____

_____

_____

_____

_____

_____

_____

_____

BIRTH EXPERIENCE REFLECTION SECTION 3: SPENDING TIME WITH YOUR BABY (OR BABIES)

What a journey so far. Other than perhaps through a prenatal scan, this is the first time you are laying eyes on your baby (or babies). This is not always a time of pure happiness; you might have mixed feelings. Maybe there is some lingering fear or anxiety. Maybe you are neck-deep in awe. Maybe the grief you feel is bigger than any words. It's all okay. Remember: This is your story. No one can tell you your feelings are out of place. You're safe.

One

What were your first thoughts after your baby was (or babies were) born?

_____

_____

_____

_____

_____

_____

_____

_____

_____

_____

_____

_____

_____

_____

_____

_____

Two

Which emotions were present for you at this time? No judgment is needed; you felt what you felt. Remember: Many mixed feelings can show up all at the same time, or perhaps there is one super-loud emotion. Was this how you thought you might feel after birth?

_____

_____

_____

_____

_____

_____

_____

_____

_____

_____

_____

_____

_____

Three

Do you remember any physical sensations? Were you able, or did you want, to see and touch your baby (or babies) right away? How did your body feel? How did their body (or bodies) feel? If your baby was (or babies were) living, did you have any thoughts about what your baby (or babies) might be thinking or feeling?

_____

_____

_____

_____

_____

_____

_____

_____

_____

_____

_____

_____

_____

_____

Four

What feels sacred about these first moments with your baby (or babies)? If nothing does, that's okay. Reflect on that, too. Did anything feel out of place?

_____

_____

_____

_____

_____

_____

_____

_____

_____

_____

_____

_____

_____

Five

Were the first post-birth moments what you expected? How did they feel different? How did they feel aligned? See if you can let in some gentleness about any misalignment.

_____

_____

_____

_____

_____

_____

_____

_____

_____

_____

_____

_____

_____

After this section you may, when you're ready, want to move directly to the next Birth Experience Reflection section, Section 4: Stillbirth Reflection. Or, your story may travel next to Birth Experience Reflection Section 5: After. See what feels best, and go there. If you need more space for journaling, don't forget there are some extra lined pages at the end of each section.

Other Thoughts

_____

_____

_____

_____

_____

_____

_____

_____

_____

_____

_____

_____

_____

_____

_____

_____

Other Thoughts

Other Thoughts

_____

_____

_____

_____

_____

_____

_____

_____

_____

_____

_____

_____

_____

_____

_____

_____

BIRTH EXPERIENCE REFLECTION SECTION 4: STILLBIRTH REFLECTION

This section is for reflecting on being with your baby (or babies) after they were born, when they had already passed. This tender time can look very different from experience to experience, and so there is plenty of space here for reflecting on how this time looked for you.

One

How much space were you given to just be with your baby (or babies)? Did you want to see them? What about touch them? Did holding them feel right to you? If you held your baby (or babies), how did their body feel? In what ways did they look the same or different than how you imagined they would?

_____

_____

_____

_____

_____

_____

_____

_____

_____

_____

_____

_____

_____

_____

_____

Two

How did your providers speak with you after the birth of your baby (or babies)? How did they interact with your baby (or babies)?

Three

In what ways was your baby (or were your babies) cared for? Did this feel respectful to you? Did you feel that they were being shown love?

_____

_____

_____

_____

_____

_____

_____

_____

_____

_____

_____

_____

_____

_____

_____

_____

_____

Four

Did you have the opportunity for photos to be taken of your baby (or babies), or of you and your baby (or babies)? If so, is that something you decided to do? Reflect on your decision-making around this. Did you want photos to be part of how you would remember your little one(s)? What were your unique ways of creating memories with them other than photos? Did any of your providers play a role in helping you find ways to create memories or give you guidance on what to do with your baby (or babies)?

_____

_____

_____

_____

_____

_____

_____

_____

_____

_____

_____

_____

Five

Were there things you were able to tell your baby (or babies), either aloud or in your mind?

_____

_____

_____

_____

_____

_____

_____

_____

_____

_____

_____

_____

_____

_____

_____

_____

_____

Six

This space is for an outpouring of all the words you felt while being with your baby (or babies) after their birth—*all* of the words: the big ones, the loud ones, the angry ones, the sweet ones, the quiet ones. Let all of them be here together. It's all allowed. See if you can breathe in a bit of opening in just letting these all exist at once. Remember: Having emotional complexity is part of being human.

_____

_____

_____

_____

_____

_____

_____

_____

_____

_____

_____

_____

_____

When you're ready, turn the page. More reflection awaits. If you need more space for journaling, don't forget there are some extra lined pages at the end of each section.

Other Thoughts

_____

_____

_____

_____

_____

_____

_____

_____

_____

_____

_____

_____

_____

_____

_____

_____

_____

Other Thoughts

_____

_____

_____

_____

_____

_____

_____

_____

_____

_____

_____

_____

_____

_____

Other Thoughts

_____

_____

_____

_____

_____

_____

_____

_____

_____

_____

_____

_____

_____

_____

_____

BIRTH EXPERIENCE REFLECTION SECTION 5: AFTER

Your story doesn't end after your birth experience. There is still so much more to say. In the hours, days, and weeks after this life-shifting time, deep adjustment and transformation happen. You see, you have just been birthed as a parent as well—for the first time or even the fifth time. Even if your baby is (or babies are) not present with you, you experienced this shift. This section gives you an opportunity to stand toward the tail end of your birth story, looking back at themes and the whole picture. By the end of this section, you will have an opportunity to name your story.

One

In the moments after a baby is (or babies are) born, you can experience a wide variety of scenarios. Let's talk about expectations. Our vision of something, before we experience it, can be vastly different from the reality of living it. What were your expectations of birth (how it would feel, how you would experience it, how those around you would act, etc.)? How did these expectations differ from reality? Are there any of these differences that are ready to move or be released?

_____

_____

_____

_____

_____

_____

_____

_____

_____

_____

_____

_____

Two

Similarly, what beliefs did you have about birth before going through it? For example, did you believe birth "should" be a certain way? Or that a certain type of birth or choice meant something about you? How, if at all, has your perspective changed?

_____

_____

_____

_____

_____

_____

_____

_____

_____

_____

_____

_____

_____

_____

Three

Who was around you in the moments and days following birth? How did this environment feel? In what ways were you being supported, and in what ways did you need to be supported?

Four

What highlights do you have around your birth story? When might you have felt empowered? Strong? When your story is laced with grief, it might feel odd to answer this question. Be gentle. When you're ready, though, you might be able to point to times when you showed strength or other similar qualities in your story.

_____

_____

_____

_____

_____

_____

_____

_____

_____

_____

_____

_____

_____

Five

Look within yourself. Are you holding any feelings of regret? Where are they lingering in your story?

_____

_____

_____

_____

_____

_____

_____

_____

_____

_____

_____

_____

_____

_____

_____

_____

Six

Reflect on your feelings about your body. How did you feel about your body right after birth? How do you feel about it now? What has changed? What has remained the same? Our bodies stretch, shift, and change, and they can show up for us in innumerable ways. It is possible to honor your body in both its imperfections and in its capabilities.

_____

_____

_____

_____

_____

_____

_____

_____

_____

_____

_____

_____

_____

_____

Seven

Choose some words to describe your birth story, after you've taken time to reflect. It's okay if you don't feel all of them are positive. It's your story, and it's real, and it's all allowed.

_____

_____

_____

_____

_____

_____

_____

_____

_____

_____

_____

_____

_____

_____

Eight

If you were to choose a title for your birth story, what would it be? Go with whatever feels right. Would there be a certain image, experience, or memory that you highlight here? Or is there a feeling you'd like to focus on? Your story's title is allowed to be whatever you want.

_____

_____

_____

_____

_____

_____

_____

_____

_____

_____

_____

_____

_____

_____

_____

_____

Nine

Is there an epilogue to your birth story? Think about what might be presented in this section. Carry this forward. Think about how you will relay your baby's (or babies') birth story from now on. What will you choose to tell family members and others in your life? What will you tell yourself?

If you experienced a NICU stay with your little one(s), turn the page when you're ready. Otherwise, you may wish to visit the Infant Loss Reflection section or keep moving along to the Remembering and Honoring Your Baby (or Babies) section. Go at your own pace, and be gentle with yourself. If you need more space for journaling, don't forget there are some extra lined pages at the end of each section.

Other Thoughts

Other Thoughts

Other Thoughts

_____

_____

_____

_____

_____

_____

_____

_____

_____

_____

_____

_____

_____

_____

_____

_____

NICU STAY REFLECTION

A NICU experience is many times, though not always, unexpected. Talking about expectations, this can be a wild departure from the vision you may have been imagining. This section is here for you to spend some time with your little one's (or little ones') extended hospital stay. Even though they were likely the focus of care, your experience is also deeply important.

One

Did you feel prepared for your baby's (or babies') NICU stay? In which ways did you feel accepting, and in which ways did you feel caught off guard?

_____

_____

_____

_____

_____

_____

_____

_____

_____

_____

_____

_____

_____

_____

_____

_____

Two

What was the NICU environment like for you? What did it actually feel like to your physical body? Who else was around, and in what ways did they help this process (or not)?

_____

_____

_____

_____

_____

_____

_____

_____

_____

_____

_____

_____

_____

_____

_____

Three

What were the biggest challenges of spending time in the NICU?

_____

_____

_____

_____

_____

_____

_____

_____

_____

_____

_____

_____

_____

_____

_____

_____

_____

Four

What were the unexpected gifts that came from spending time in the NICU?

_____

_____

_____

_____

_____

_____

_____

_____

_____

_____

_____

_____

_____

_____

_____

_____

_____

Five

What did you learn about yourself as a result of being with your baby (or babies) in the NICU? If a partner was part of this story, what did you learn about them? What did you learn about your baby (or babies)?

_____

_____

_____

_____

_____

_____

_____

_____

_____

_____

_____

_____

_____

_____

_____

Six

Notice what, if anything, might need to be forgiven, specifically around the time spent in the NICU. Some parents hold a sense of responsibility about things they could have done differently or may have some feelings, such as anger, toward a situation or a provider. What's present for you? Is any amount of this ready to be released? Sometimes our releases happen in degrees, not all at once. Bit by bit, we begin to heal. You are healing.

Infant Loss Reflection is the next section. When you're ready, see if it feels right to move there next. Take your time. This space is for you, so you make the rules and set the pace. If you need more space for journaling, don't forget there are some extra lined pages at the end of each section.

Other Thoughts

_____

_____

_____

_____

_____

_____

_____

_____

_____

_____

_____

_____

_____

_____

_____

Other Thoughts

Other Thoughts

_____

_____

_____

_____

_____

_____

_____

_____

_____

_____

_____

_____

_____

_____

_____

INFANT LOSS REFLECTION

There is a range of time people have with their babies while they are living. Whether it was a matter of hours, days, weeks, or months, you have space here to reflect on the end of your little one's life (or little ones' lives). Your birth experience matters. The time with them matters. Your feelings matter. Your story matters.

One

How did it feel to begin a parenting journey with your little one (or little ones)? What were the most memorable parts?

_____

_____

_____

_____

_____

_____

_____

_____

_____

_____

_____

_____

_____

_____

Two

Were there aspects of your baby's (or babies') personality or temperament that stood out to you? What were they? It's possible that these showed up for you intuitively; even if you did not have much time with your baby (or babies), it's possible that you felt an inner knowing about them. Reflect on the ways your baby (or babies) showed who they were.

_____

_____

_____

_____

_____

_____

_____

_____

_____

_____

_____

_____

_____

_____

Three

What early memories are sacred to you? Are there any that feel especially warm?

_____

_____

_____

_____

_____

_____

_____

_____

_____

_____

_____

_____

_____

_____

_____

Four

It is common for some memories to be tinged with regret. See if there might be the tiniest bit of room for self-compassion. If you're not sure where to start, try imagining a friend telling you about the memory as if it were their own. How would you respond to them? What types of comfort might you offer?

_____

_____

_____

_____

_____

_____

_____

_____

_____

_____

_____

_____

_____

Five

Was the loss of your baby (or babies) something you knew may happen ahead of time? Nothing can prepare you for that loss. How did you cope with knowing you may not have much time left with your baby (or babies)?

_____

_____

_____

_____

_____

_____

_____

_____

_____

_____

_____

_____

_____

_____

Six

In what ways were you able to say goodbye to your baby (or babies), even if this couldn't happen when or how you wanted? Were there certain actions you took, like writing a letter or visiting a specific spot in nature? Or was this something that involved physical touch with your baby (or babies)? While saying goodbye in any form might not have felt welcome, reflect on how it happened and how it aligned with, or did not align with, your hopes.

_____

_____

_____

_____

_____

_____

_____

_____

_____

_____

_____

_____

_____

_____

Seven

Where did your baby (or babies) pass away? Were you present at the time? Who was with you? Was anyone able to hold you, physically or otherwise?

_____

_____

_____

_____

_____

_____

_____

_____

_____

_____

_____

_____

_____

_____

_____

_____

Eight

In what ways was your baby (or were your babies) cared for after they passed away? Did this feel respectful to you? Were you able to spend time with your little one (or little ones)? What were your thoughts? Fears? Questions?

_____

_____

_____

_____

_____

_____

_____

_____

_____

_____

_____

_____

_____

_____

_____

Other Thoughts

Other Thoughts

Other Thoughts

_____

_____

_____

_____

_____

_____

_____

_____

_____

_____

_____

_____

_____

_____

_____

_____

REMEMBERING AND HONORING YOUR BABY (OR BABIES)

This section is to reflect on your baby (or babies) and what lies ahead. Again, perhaps the word *"baby"* doesn't resonate with you—that's okay, just use the word that does. Be gentle as you travel through this section, taking breaks as needed and returning when it feels right. If it feels aligned for you, take a deep breath here and send some love to your little one(s). See it traveling to them and turn the page when you're ready.

One

Did you name your baby (or babies)? What is your baby's name (or babies' names)? Reflect on the meaning or story behind their name (or names), and how it feels in your body when you say it out loud or to yourself. Where do you feel it within? If you have not named your baby (or babies) yet, it's not too late—if it's something that feels right. If it does, tune in to the energy of your baby (or babies). Their name doesn't need to be a traditional name; it could be anything.

Two

If you were able to see your baby (or babies) prior to them passing, what did they look like? What was most memorable to you about them? Did they remind you of anyone?

_____

_____

_____

_____

_____

_____

_____

_____

_____

_____

_____

_____

_____

_____

Three

If you were not able to see your baby (or babies) prior to them passing, did you imagine what they might look like? How did they appear in your mind's eye?

Four

In what way(s) was your baby (or were your babies) honored by your providers? How did this sit with you? Was anything missing? What, if anything, do you wish they had done differently?

_____

_____

_____

_____

_____

_____

_____

_____

_____

_____

_____

_____

_____

_____

_____

Five

Did you and/or your family have an event or do something in particular to remember your baby (or babies)? What did you do? Was this what you wanted to do? What feelings are you holding about how your ideal event did or did not align with what happened?

_____

_____

_____

_____

_____

_____

_____

_____

_____

_____

_____

_____

_____

_____

_____

_____

Six

What do you most want your baby (or babies) to know? This could be how you feel about them, things you wanted to teach them, or anything else.

_____

_____

_____

_____

_____

_____

_____

_____

_____

_____

_____

_____

_____

_____

_____

_____

Seven

Does your baby (or babies) share messages with you? Some people may find a connection with their little one by seeing things such as a particular type of bird or coin, or hearing a specific song.

_____

_____

_____

_____

_____

_____

_____

_____

_____

_____

_____

_____

_____

_____

Eight

In which ways have you been allowed to grieve? In which ways do you still need to grieve? Grief is fluid and flows. It can feel alive, all-consuming sometimes and a bit less loud at other times. How will you create space for your grief when it needs to have a voice?

_____

_____

_____

_____

_____

_____

_____

_____

_____

_____

_____

_____

_____

_____

Nine

Do you have a way to communicate to those around you that you are having a big grief day or moment? Or that you are really thinking about your baby (or babies) at that time? That might even be a way of showing that the feeling is present, even if it means you don't feel like talking about it.

Ten

What anticipated futures are you grieving? This could mean things you envisioned such as having playground adventures, exploring the world, or even watching your baby's (or babies') first steps. These can be very simple things, or much bigger dreams.

_____

_____

_____

_____

_____

_____

_____

_____

_____

_____

_____

_____

_____

_____

_____

Eleven

In what ways do you envision partnering with your baby (or babies) moving forward? This could be taking action around a specific cause, or even something so quiet as feeling them with you as you go about your day in compassion and love.

_____

_____

_____

_____

_____

_____

_____

_____

_____

_____

_____

_____

_____

_____

Twelve

Moving forward, what is the story you will tell yourself about your baby (or babies)? What will you tell others? Feel this story in your body and radiating beyond. Allow yourself to just be with it. You have done so much important reflection.

_____

_____

_____

_____

_____

_____

_____

_____

_____

_____

_____

_____

_____

_____

Other Thoughts

Other Thoughts

Other Thoughts

_____

_____

_____

_____

_____

_____

_____

_____

_____

_____

_____

_____

_____

_____

_____

_____

BE IN YOUR BODY

We have spent a great deal of time in a place of reflection. Sometimes that can take us deeply into our minds and thoughts, thereby leaving the body behind, though my aim was to keep your body involved in this process as well. Let's take some time now to reconnect with your physical self.

Bring your hand to your chest, over your heart. If that doesn't feel comfortable, see what does. Maybe placing one hand over the other in your lap feels supportive, or maybe placing a hand on your belly does. Tap it there several times, just lightly, or stretch your fingers. See if your body feels the need for some gentle movement. Invite in some stretching or rocking side to side. Whatever feels right to you, let it be.

Being with your body may feel unfamiliar. That is absolutely okay. Say hello to it. Know that in some ways you are just getting to know each other, and in other ways there is a long, shared history. See if you might be open to beginning to write a new story with your body, now.

Give yourself permission to be in this body. Allow this body the opportunity to serve you, even if in ways that so far are mysterious. Be curious. Welcome forgiveness if needed.

And in the end, remember this: You are human. You are figuring things out. You are living.

GRATITUDE

Thank you for spending this time with your birth and loss stories. I am so glad you chose to explore this part of yourself and your life. Thank you for letting me walk this path with you. Honor your story as a powerful experience, one of the many pieces that will come together to shape who you are becoming. Let it propel you forward when it's time to take action, and let it hold you when you need to be held. Don't let this book be the end of your exploration, either. Keep this momentum going. You will be given many opportunities for growth and advancement, so don't be afraid to listen when they speak to you.

ACKNOWLEDGMENTS

As with all of my projects, books and otherwise, it would have been impossible for this book to come into being without a great deal of support. These supports show up in all different ways, and I am grateful for each of them. Friends gave words of encouragement when my confidence or energy was waning, and my husband listened time and time again as I processed my thoughts out loud. I want to give specific thanks for these individuals as well:

Beta Readers

To Kerri-Anne, Ren, Jessie, and Sadija—thank you so much for taking time out of your lives to provide invaluable feedback about the flow and content of this book! I value each of your lived experiences, and I feel fortunate each of you shared your wisdom with me.

Foreword Authors

To Betsy and Kiley—I am so grateful you believed in this project and share my love for the importance of story. The work that you both do is amazing and serves so many. Thank you for bringing your experience into the foreword, sharing such compassionate words with readers, and giving helpful feedback about the book.

Editing

To Jodi—you did it again! When we first met, I had no idea we would have the opportunity to work on multiple projects together and am so glad my path has pointed to writing projects again and again. You are such a delight to work with and give me the exact type of support I need. Thank you!

Design

To Jess—thank you for bringing your skills and vision into this project! It is a breeze to work with you and I love seeing how you create an experience for readers using design. I feel so lucky to have you on my team!

ABOUT THE AUTHOR

Emily Souder is a licensed clinical social worker certified in perinatal mental health, an intuitive guide, and a Reiki master practitioner. She and her family live in Maryland, homeschooling and exploring, and getting curious about life. Emily loves tea, finding mushrooms in the woods, and drawing amusement from where she can.

Emily has written multiple books, including *Birth Story Brave, Re-imagined: A Guide for Reflecting on Your Childbirth Experience* and *Sparks: Inspiration for Extinguishing the Power of Fear and Igniting Amusement, Knowing, and Trust*.

Learn more at www.emilysouder.com.

Made in the USA
Middletown, DE
16 October 2023